NO DIVORCE

A HAPPY HOME FOREVER

By

Joni Jackson

Table Of Contents

INTRODUCTIONS

Marriage is an institution that has been around for centuries, and it remains an essential part of human society today. However, in recent times, the rate of divorce has risen significantly, and it is becoming increasingly common for marriages to end in separation. This trend is worrying, and it highlights the need for couples to understand the secrets to a happy home without divorce.

"No Divorce: A Happy Home Forever" is a book that aims to provide couples with the tools and strategies they need to build a happy and lasting marriage. The book is written by experts who have years of experience working with couples and helping them navigate the challenges of married life.

The book is designed to be a practical guide that couples can use to build a stronger and more fulfilling marriage. It covers a wide range of topics, including communication, conflict resolution, familiarity, and parenting. The authors of the book understand that every couple is unique, and they provide practical advice that can be customized to fit the needs of each module.

The book is divided into several chapters, each of which focuses on a specific aspect of marriage. The first chapter is an introduction to the book and sets the stage for what is to come. It provides an overview of the topics that will be covered in the book and highlights the importance of building a happy home without divorce.

The second chapter focuses on communication, which is one of the most critical elements of a successful marriage. The authors provide practical tips on how couples can communicate effectively and avoid common communication pitfalls.
To show you how important communication is in every chapter of this book you will come across the word communication.

The third chapter is about conflict resolution, which is another critical aspect of a happy marriage. The authors provide strategies that couples can use to resolve conflicts in a healthily active fourth chapter is about intimacy, which is a vital component of a fulfilling marriage. The authors provide tips on how couples can build intimacy and keep the spark alive in their relationship.

The fifth chapter is about parenting, which is another significant challenge that many couples face. The authors provide practical advice on how couples can work together to raise happy and healthy children.

The final chapter of the book is a conclusion that brings everything together. has summarised the key points of the book and provides a roadmap for couples who want to build a happy home without divorce.

In conclusion, "No Divorce Happy Home Forever" is an essential guide for couples who want to build a strong and lasting marriage. The book provides practical advice that can be customized to fit the needs of each individual. It is an invaluable resource for anyone who wants to build a happy home without divorce.

CHAPTER 1 Building a Strong Foundation:

Building a strong foundation is critical for any relationship to thrive. Among the many key factors that contribute to the success of a relationship, communication, and trust are two of the most essential elements. They are the building blocks that lay the groundwork for a healthy and fulfilling relationship. In this essay, we will discuss the importance of communication and trust in relationships and the various ways in which they can be developed and strengthened.

Communication is the foundation of any relationship. It is how we convey our thoughts, feelings, and ideas to one another. Effective communication is essential for building trust, resolving conflicts, and fostering intimacy in a relationship. Communication can take many forms, including oral, nonoral, and written communication. Each form has its advantages and disadvantages, but all are important for building strong relationships.

Oral communication is the most common form of communication. It includes spoken words, tone of voice, and inflection. Verbal communication is important because it allows us to express our thoughts and feelings directly to our partners. It also allows us to receive feedback and understand our partner's thoughts and feelings. When we communicate verbally, we should always be clear, concise, and Respectful. It is also important to actively listen to our partners and show empathy toward their feelings.

Nonorall communication is another important form of communication. It includes body language, facial expressions, and gestures. Nonverbal communication can convey messages that words cannot, and it is often more honest than verbal communication. For example, a person may say that they are delighted, but their body may indicate otherwise. Non-Oral communication can be a powerful tool for building trust and understanding in a relationship. However, it is important to be aware of our nonverbal cues and to interpret our partner's nonverbal cues accurately.

Written communication is another important form of communication. It includes text messages, emails, and letters. Written communication can be useful for expressing Complex thoughts and feelings that may be difficult to communicate verbally. It can also be a useful tool for resolving conflicts and clarifying misunderstandings. However, written communication can be misinterpreted, and it is important to be clear and concise when communicating in writing.

Trust is another essential component of a strong foundation in a relationship. Trust is built over time through consistent activities and behaviors that illustrate reliability, truthfulness, and innocence. Trust is the foundation for intimacy and vulnerability in a relationship. Without trust, a relationship cannot thrive.

To build trust in a relationship, it is important to be honest, and transparent with your partner. This means being honest about your opinions, emotions, and efforts. It also implies being trustworthy and keeping your commitments. It is important to Communicate openly and to avoid keeping secrets from your partner. Trust is built through consistency, so it is important to demonstrate reliable and trustworthy behavior over time.

Trust can also be built by showing empathy and understanding toward your partner's feelings and needs. This means listening actively, showing empathy, and responding to your partner's needs with care and compassion. It is important to be sensitive to your partner's feelings and to avoid dismissive or critical responses.

In addition to communication and trust, other important factors contribute to a strong foundation in a relationship. These include mutual respect, shared values and goals, and a willingness to compromise and work through conflicts together. When both partners are committed to building a strong foundation in their relationship, they can Overcome challenges and build a lasting and fulfilling partnership.

In conclusion, communication and trust are essential components of a strong foundation in any relationship. Effective communication allows us to express our thoughts and feelings, resolve conflicts, and foster intimacy. Trust is

built through consistent actions and conducts that
demonstrate reliability, honesty, and integrity.
By prioritizing communication, trust, and other important
factors, couples can build a strong foundation that supports
Being open to change, embracing new ideas, and
proactively responding to challenges allow individuals to
remain agile and stay ahead of the curve. A strong
foundation is built on the ability to navigate uncertainties
and bounce back from setbacks.

Discipline and Consistency:
Discipline and consistency are essential habits that
contribute to a strong foundation in relationships. The
ability to maintain focus, adhere to schedules, and follow
through on commitments instills a sense of reliability and
trustworthiness. Consistent effort and discipline create a
stable framework upon which progress can be made,
fostering long-term growth and success.

Emotional Intelligence:
Emotional intelligence plays a significant role in building a
strong foundation in relationships. Understanding and
managing one's emotions, as well as empathizing with
others, enhances interpersonal relationships and promotes
effective teamwork. Emotional intelligence fosters a
positive and supportive environment, reinforcing the
foundation of trust and collaboration.

Strategic Thinking:
Strategic thinking is a vital skill for building a strong
foundation relationship. It involves analyzing situations,
considering multiple perspectives, and making decisions
that align with long-term goals. Strategic thinkers
anticipate challenges, identify opportunities, and
proactively plan for the future, ensuring a solid foundation
that can withstand external pressures.

 Accountability and Responsibility:
Taking accountability and being responsible for one's
actions and decisions is integral to building a strong
foundation. Being accountable fosters trust and credibility,
as it demonstrates reliability and integrity. Individuals and
organizations that take ownership of their responsibilities
create a stable foundation upon which others can rely.

 Collaboration and Teamwork:
Collaboration and teamwork are essential elements in
building a strong foundation in relationships. By fostering
an environment where diverse perspectives are valued,
individuals can harness the collective intelligence and
strengths of their teams.

CHAPTER 2 Navigating Conflicts:

Conflict is an inevitable part of human interplay. It can arise in any place, whether or not at home, within the place of a job, or at social gatherings. Conflicts get up when people have divergent hobbies, evaluations, or values, and they understand that their goals are being threatened. If no longer controlled properly, conflicts can boost and result in bad consequences, consisting of broken relationships, decreased productivity, or even violence. Therefore, it's far important to have effective strategies for resolving disagreements. In this article, we will discuss various methods of navigating Conflicts, which include verbal exchange strategies, hassle-fixing techniques, negotiation techniques, and mediation techniques.

Communication Techniques

Effective communique is the muse for resolving conflicts. People should be able to specify their thoughts and emotions without a doubt and listen actively to others' views. However, many conflicts arise because of miscommunication or loss of communique. Therefore, it's far important to develop top conversation capabilities, which include:

Active Listening: Active listening involves paying close attention to what the alternative person is announcing, asking clarifying questions, and reflecting on what you have heard to ensure you recognize their attitude.

Using "I" Statements: "I" statements are a way of expressing your emotions without accusing or blaming others. For example, in preference to announcing, "You always interrupt me," say, "I feel annoyed once I am interrupted."

Avoiding Trigger Words: Some phrases or terms can trigger negative reactions and expand conflicts. For instance, the usage of phrases like "constantly" and "by no means" can sound accusatory and make people defensive.

Summarizing: Summarizing involves paraphrasing the alternative character's key factors to show that you have understood their attitude. This method can assist avoid misunderstandings and clarify the problems at hand.

Problem-Solving Methods

Another approach to navigating conflicts is the consciousness of finding a jointly beneficial approach to the problem. This technique involves figuring out the root causes of the struggle, brainstorming ability answers, and comparing the pros and cons of every choice. The following hassle-fixing methods can assist remedy disagreements:

Identify the Problem: The first step in hassle-solving is to discover the unique difficulty inflicting warfare. It is critical to be unique and keep away from generalizations or assumptions.

Brainstorm Solutions: Once the problem has been recognized, brainstorming viable answers is the next step. All events involved Ought to make contributions to their ideas without judgment.

Evaluate Solutions: After producing a list of capacity answers, evaluate each option's professionals and cons. It is important to don't forget the impact of each solution on all parties involved.

Choose a Solution: Finally, pick out the solution that fine meets the wishes of all events involved. It is essential to communicate the selection truly and ensure that everybody is aware of the selected answer.

Negotiation Tactics

Negotiation is a process of dialogue aimed toward attaining an agreement that satisfies all of us's pastimes. Negotiation can be an Effective tool for resolving conflicts when there's no apparent solution. Negotiation includes the following techniques:

Find Common Ground: The first step in negotiation is to discover shared pastimes or values. This can assist establish a sense of trust and know-how between the events involved.

Identify Differences: Once the ot-unusual ground has been mounted, it's miles essential to perceive the regions wherein the parties disagree. This can assist make clear the specific troubles that need to be addressed.

Brainstorm Solutions: Brainstorming potential solutions is the next step in negotiation. It is critical to hold an open mind and be willing to recall a diffusion of alternatives.

Make Concessions: Negotiation frequently involves making concessions or compromises. It is vital to be bendy and willing to make trade-offs to attain an agreement.

Mediation Strategies

Mediation is a process wherein a neutral 0.33 birthday celebration helps the parties involved in a battle attain and at the same time desirable

Disagreements in marriage are inevitable, and it is how couples clear up these variations which can make or damage their courting. When people come collectively to form a union, it is nearly not possible to agree on the whole lot. At a few points, disagreements will stand up, and how couples navigate these conflicts is crucial to Retaining a wholesome and successful marriage. In this newsletter, we're going to speak about some techniques for resolving disagreements in marriage.

Firstly, it is important to keep in mind that war is normal in any dating, and it's no longer always an awful aspect. Disagreements can frequently result in more information and can toughen a pair's bond. It's vital to approach disagreements with open thoughts and a willingness to compromise. Often, the solution to a problem lies somewhere inside the center, and each companion wan wants to be willing to provide a little to solve it.

Effective communication is important in resolving disagreements. When discussing a problem, both partners should take turns expressing their minds and feelings without Interrupting or brushing off the alternative man or woman's attitude. It's essential to pay attention actively and to attempt to understand where the alternative individual is coming from. Sometimes, just feeling heard can be sufficient to remedy a disagreement.

Another essential strategy for resolving disagreements is to awareness of the hassle, now not the character. It's clean to turn out to be protecting while our reviews are challenged, but it's crucial to keep in mind that the problem to hand is the problem, not the person. Couples should avoid attacking each other for my part and as a substitute cognizance of finding a strategy for the hassle to hand. Using "I" statements rather than "you" statements may be a useful manner to express worries without setting blame on the other individual.

Compromise is frequently vital to clear up disagreements in marriage. Both companions want to be inclined to give a bit to discover an answer that works for each of them. Compromise doesn't suggest that one individual wins and the other loses; it approaches locating a solution that satisfies both companions' needs. It's critical to take into account that compromise is a two-way street, and each partner needs to be willing to present and take.

It's also important to pick the proper time and vicinity to talk about disagreements. Bringing up contentious trouble in the course of a busy workday or in front of others can strengthen the scenario and make it easier to discover a decision. Couples must set aside time to talk about issues in a non-public place where they can be conscious of locating an answer without distractions.

In a few cases, it can be necessary to seek outside help to solve a confrontation. Couples remedy can be a beneficial tool for couples who are struggling to clear up conflicts on their own. An educated therapist can provide objective insights and techniques to help couples find a decision that works for each partner.

Disagreements in marriage are inevitable, and the way couples take care of these conflicts is essential to keeping a healthy and successful date. Effective communication, a focus on the hassle rather than the person, compromise, and choosing the proper time and location to talk about troubles are all essential strategies for resolving disagreements. When disagreements end up too hard to solve on their very own, searching for outdoor assistance from a therapist may be a useful device for finding a decision. By approaching disagreements with an open mind, a willingness to compromise, and a focus on locating a solution that works for both companions, couples can improve their bond and maintain a satisfied and wholesome marriage

8 ULTIMATE STEPS TO CONSIDER

1 Active Listening: Active listening is a fundamental skill that underpins successful conflict resolution. It involves giving your full attention to the other person, understanding their perspective, and validating their feelings. By actively listening, you demonstrate empathy and create an atmosphere of open communication, which fosters productive dialogue and problem-solving.

2. Effective Communication: Clear and assertive communication is crucial when addressing conflicts in relationships. Express your thoughts and concerns using "I" statements, which focus on your feelings and experiences rather than placing blame on the other person. This approach encourages mutual understanding and avoids escalating tensions.

3. Respect and Empathy: Treating each other with respect and empathy is vital during conflicts. Remember that individuals have different viewpoints and experiences that shape their perspectives. Show empathy by attempting to understand the other person's feelings and needs. This can help build rapport and trust, laying the foundation for finding common ground.

4. Collaborative Problem-Solving: Instead of approaching conflicts as win-lose scenarios, strive for collaborative

problem-solving. Seek mutually beneficial solutions by exploring different alternatives and brainstorming together. Encourage creativity and open-mindedness to find innovative approaches that address the concerns of all parties involved.

5. Focus on Interests, not Positions: Often, conflicts arise from differing positions on a particular issue. Instead of fixating on positions, delve deeper into the underlying interests and needs of each party. By understanding the motivations and desires driving each person, it becomes easier to identify creative solutions that satisfy everyone involved.

6. Time and Place: Choosing the right time and place for conflict resolution is crucial. Ensure that both parties are in a calm state of mind and that the environment is conducive to open communication. Avoid public settings or situations where interruptions are likely. By setting the stage appropriately, you enhance the chances of a constructive conversation.

7. Seek Mediation if Necessary: In some cases, conflicts in relationships may reach an impasse, making it challenging to resolve them without external intervention. If direct communication proves ineffective, consider involving a neutral third party, such as a professional mediator or

counselor. These professionals possess the expertise to facilitate constructive discussions and help guide the process toward a resolution.

8. Learn from the Experience: Conflict offers an opportunity for growth and learning. After a conflict has been resolved, take time to reflect on the experience. Identify areas for personal improvement, such as communication skills or emotional intelligence. Use the conflict as a stepping stone for self-development, aiming to enhance your ability to navigate future conflicts successfully.

Navigating conflicts in relationships requires a professional approach that prioritizes active listening, effective communication, respect, empathy, collaborative problem-solving, and a focus on interests rather than positions. By employing these strategies, individuals can enhance their conflict resolution skills and foster healthier, more resilient relationships. Remember, conflicts are not necessarily detrimental; when managed effectively, they can lead to stronger connections and personal growth

CHAPTER 3 Balancing Responsibilities:

In today's fast-paced world, juggling multiple responsibilities has become a norm for most people, especially for those who are parents. Raising children and managing a household require significant amounts of time, energy, and resources, leaving little room for personal or professional pursuits. While men and women have come a long way in achieving gender equality, there remains a significant imbalance in the division of household chores and parenting duties. This paper will explore the various factors that contribute to the unequal distribution of responsibilities, the consequences of such an imbalance, and strategies for achieving a fair and balanced division of household and parenting duties.

Factors Contributing to the Unequal Division of Household Chores and Parenting Duties

Several factors contribute to the unequal distribution of household chores and parenting duties. Some of these factors include:

Traditional Gender Roles: Despite the progress made in achieving gender equality, traditional gender roles persist in many societies. Women are still seen as the primary caregivers and homemakers, while men are expected to be the breadwinners. These gender roles are deeply entrenched in society and often influence how couples divide their responsibilities.

Unequal Workload: Studies have shown that women perform a disproportionate amount of household chores and parenting duties, even when both partners work outside the home. This is because women are expected to bear the primary responsibility for childcare and domestic work, even when they are employed full-time.

Lack of Communication: Communication is key to any successful relationship, and this is no different when it comes to dividing household and parenting responsibilities. Often, couples fail to communicate their expectations and needs, leading to misunderstandings and resentment.

Unconscious Bias: Sometimes, couples may not even be aware that they are perpetuating gender stereotypes and biases. This could be because they have internalized these beliefs and attitudes, or because they are not aware of the impact that their actions are having on their partner.

Consequences of an Imbalance in Household and Parenting Duties

An imbalance in household and parenting duties can have several negative consequences for both partners and their children. Some of these consequences include:

Stress and Burnout: When one partner is responsible for the majority of the household and parenting duties, they may experience higher levels of stress and burnout. This can lead to physical and mental health problems, which can impact their ability to parent effectively.

Relationship Problems: An imbalance in household and parenting duties can strain the relationship between partners, leading to resentment, conflict, and ultimately, a breakdown in the relationship.

Inequity: An unequal distribution of responsibilities can create a sense of inequity, which can damage the self-esteem and confidence of the partner who feels they are bearing an unfair burden.

Negative Impact on Children: Children are also affected by an imbalance in household and parenting duties. They may feel neglected or unsupported, which can impact their emotional and social development.

Strategies for Achieving a Fair and Balanced Division of Household and Parenting Duties

Achieving a fair and balanced division of household and parenting duties requires a concerted effort from both partners. Some strategies for achieving this include:

Communication: Communication is key to any successful relationship, and this is no different when it comes to dividing household and parenting responsibilities. Couples should openly discuss their expectations, needs, and concerns, and work together to find solutions that work for both partners.

Sharing the Workload: Both partners should take an active role in household and parenting duties. This could involve dividing tasks based on skill or preference or taking turns doing certain tasks.

Flexibility: Flexibility is crucial when it comes to balancing responsibilities. Partners should be willing to adjust their schedules and routines to accommodate each other's needs and responsibilities.

Delegating Responsibilities: Partners should be willing to delegate

CHAPTER 4: Maintaining Romance:

When a couple first falls in love, everything feels magical and effortless. But over time, the stresses of life can take their toll, and it's not uncommon for romances to wane. With hard work, dedication, and the right strategy, you can rekindle the spark and keep the romance alive.

This book will give you some of the most effective ways to rekindle your relationship. We'll cover a variety of strategies, from the practical to the emotional, and share tips and advice on how to implement them in your relationships. Whether you've been together for months or years, these tips will help you maintain your romance and enjoy a long and fulfilling partnership.

Prioritize communication
Communication is the foundation of a healthy relationship and essential to sustaining romance. Misunderstandings, resentments, and conflicts can arise when couples stop communicating effectively. To keep the spark going, make communication a priority in your relationship. An effective strategy is to schedule regular check-ins with your partner. Take time each week to discuss your feelings, concerns,

and hopes for the future. Use this time to actively listen to your partner, validate their feelings, and express your thoughts and feelings.

The special feelings when introduced as a wife among others, 95% of women in a relationship may feel a sense of pride, joy, or a feeling of being honored when introduced as a wife, others may not attach the same significance to the title or may have mixed emotions about it.

being introduced as a wife symbolize their commitment to their partner and their role in a recognized marital relationship. It can be seen as a way of acknowledging the partnership and bond they share with their spouse, and it can be a source of pride and happiness for them.

On the other hand, not all women may prioritize or define themselves primarily by their marital status. Some may feel that their accomplishments, professional achievements, or other aspects of their identity are more important to them than being introduced as a wife. They may prefer to be recognized for their individual qualities, talents, or contributions rather than solely for their marital status.

It's important to remember that individuals' feelings and perspectives can vary greatly when introduced as a wife. Personal values, cultural backgrounds, and individual

circumstances can all influence how a woman perceives
and responds to such introductions,
Learn to know exactly how your partner reacts when
introduced that requires sensitive action my

Another helpful tip is to practice Active Her Listening.
This means giving your conversation partner your full
attention without interrupting or defending them. It also
means repeating what you've heard to make sure his point
is correct.

make time for each other
In the hustle and bustle of everyday life, it's easy to miss
quality time with your partner. However, spending time
together is important to maintaining a strong emotional
connection and sustaining romance.

Try scheduling regular dates or weekend getaways to make
time for each other. These don't have to be expensive or
complicated. Even a quick picnic in the park or watching a
movie at home are great ways to reconnect with your loved
ones. Another effective strategy is to prioritize intimacy.
This means more than just physical intimacy (although
that's certainly important too). It also means emotional
intimacy. Take time to talk, laugh, and share experiences
with each other. This will help you feel more connected
and attuned to each other's needs and desires.

be spontaneous
One of the biggest causes of relationship stagnation is routine. Things can feel boring and unexciting when couples fall into predictable patterns of behavior.

This may mean trying new activities together, such as B. Take a dance class or going hiking. It can also mean surprising your partner with loving gestures, such as leaving a declaration of love for lunch or making your favorite food for dinner.

Every woman is like a baby
How you train the baby that's exactly who they will be coming

Express gratitude
Feeling valued is essential to maintaining a healthy and happy relationship. If your partner takes you for granted, resentment and unhappiness can creep in. Make a conscious effort to express your gratitude to your partner to keep the romance going.

This can mean thanking them for their efforts, expressing admiration for their strengths and talents, or simply telling them how much you love and appreciate them. For example, bringing a cup of coffee to bed or paying a compliment can do a lot to maintain love.

The Evolution of Romance

Romance in a relationship often changes over time. During the initial stages, there is a natural intensity and excitement that often serves as the foundation of a budding romance. However, as the relationship matures, this initial infatuation tends to subside, making it necessary for couples to actively work on maintaining the romance.

The extraordinary sentiments when presented as a spouse among Ladies. 95% of Ladies in a relationship might feel a deep satisfaction, euphoria, or a sensation of being respected when presented as a spouse, others may not connect a similar importance to the title or may have blended feelings about it.

being presented as a spouse represents their obligation to their accomplice and their part in a perceived conjugal relationship. It tends to be viewed as an approach to recognizing the organization and bond they share with their mates, and it very well may be a wellspring of pride and joy for them.

Then again, not all Ladies might focus on or characterize themselves essentially by their conjugal status. Some might feel that their achievements, proficient accomplishments, or different parts of their character mean a lot more to them than being presented as a spouse. They might like to be perceived for their singular characteristics, gifts, or commitments instead of exclusively for their conjugal status.

It's memorable's vital that people's sentiments and points of view can fluctuate incredibly when presented as a spouse.

Individual qualities, social foundations, and individual conditions can all impact how a Lady sees and answers such presentations, Figure out how to know precisely how your accomplice responds when presenting that requires delicate activity
Open and Honest Dialogue
Maintaining an open and honest dialogue is vital for sustaining romance. Couples should feel comfortable expressing their thoughts, feelings, and desires without fear of judgment or criticism. By fostering an environment of open communication, couples can address any issues that may arise, prevent misunderstandings, and promote intimacy.

Prioritizing Shared Experiences
In the hustle and bustle of everyday life, it is easy for couples to become caught up in their responsibilities.

However, prioritizing shared experiences is essential for maintaining romance. Setting aside quality time for activities that both partners enjoy can strengthen the emotional bond and create lasting memories.

Planning Date Nights
Date nights provide an opportunity for couples to reconnect and revitalize their romance. Setting aside a designated time for just the two of them, away from distractions, allows couples to focus on each other and deepen their emotional connection. Whether it's a fancy dinner, a movie night at home, or a romantic weekend getaway, date nights are essential for keeping the flame of romance alive.

Trying New Activities
Engaging in new and exciting activities together can inject fresh energy into a relationship. Exploring shared hobbies, taking up a new sport, or embarking on an adventure together fosters a sense of novelty and excitement. By stepping outside of their comfort zones and experiencing new things as a couple, partners can reignite their passion and create new avenues for romance.

CHAPTER 5 Managing External Pressures:

Stress is a common phenomenon in everyday life, and it can have a profound impact on one's health and well-being. It can also affect one's relationships, particularly marriage. External pressures, such as financial problems, job stress, and family conflicts, can strain a marriage, leading to tension and conflict. Coping with stress requires effective management of these external pressures. In this article, we will explore strategies for managing external pressures that can strain a marriage.

Recognize the Signs of Stress

One of the first steps in managing external pressures that can strain a marriage is to recognize the signs of stress. Common signs of stress include irritability, anxiety, and depression. These symptoms can manifest in different ways, such as increased arguments, lack of motivation, and changes in sleeping patterns. By recognizing these signs, couples can take steps to manage stress before it becomes overwhelming.

Set Realistic Expectations

External pressures, such as financial problems, job stress, and family conflicts, can create unrealistic expectations for couples. For example, financial difficulties can lead to unrealistic expectations about how quickly debt can be paid off, leading to tension and frustration when these expectations are not met. Similarly, job stress can create unrealistic expectations about how much time and energy one can devote to family life. Setting realistic expectations can help couples manage external pressures and avoid unnecessary tension and conflict.

Create a Supportive Environment

Creating a supportive environment is another strategy for managing external pressures that can strain a marriage. This can involve creating a comfortable and relaxing space at home, seeking support from family and friends, and engaging in activities that reduce stress, such as exercise or meditation. By creating a supportive environment, couples can better manage external pressures and avoid becoming overwhelmed.

Manage Time Effectively

Time management is another key strategy for managing external pressures that can strain a marriage. This can involve prioritizing tasks and activities, setting realistic deadlines, and delegating responsibilities when possible. Effective time management can help couples better manage external pressures and avoid becoming overwhelmed.

Maintain a Positive Outlook

Maintaining a positive outlook is another important strategy for managing external pressures that can strain a marriage. This can involve focusing on the positive aspects of one's life, such as hobbies, interests, and relationships. By maintaining a positive outlook, couples can better manage external pressures and avoid becoming overwhelmed.

Practice Self-Care

Self-care is an important aspect of managing external pressures that can strain a marriage. This can involve engaging in activities that promote physical and mental well-being, such as exercise, meditation, and self-reflection. By practicing self-care, couples can better manage external pressures and avoid becoming overwhelmed.

Seek Professional Help

In some cases, managing external pressures that can strain a marriage may require professional help. This can involve seeking counseling or therapy, either individually or as a couple. Counseling can provide couples with the tools and support they need to manage external pressures and avoid becoming overwhelmed.

Coping with stress requires effective management of external pressures that can strain a marriage. Strategies for managing external pressures include recognizing the signs of stress, setting realistic expectations, creating a supportive environment, managing time effectively, maintaining a positive outlook, practicing self-care, and seeking professional help when necessary. By adopting these strategies, couples can better manage external pressures and avoid becoming overwhelmed, leading to a stronger and more resilient marriage.

CHAPTER 6 Shared Interests and Goals:

Human beings are social creatures that thrive on connection and collaboration. Shared pursuits and desires are a critical part of constructing sturdy relationships, both private and expert. Pursuing shared pursuits and dreams creates a feeling of network, harmony, and belonging, that's crucial for our emotional and mental properly-being.

In this article, we can discover the blessings of growing together by pursuing shared pursuits and goals. We will discuss how shared interests and goals can assist people and organizations to achieve achievement, build significant relationships, and improve their usual nicely-being.

Part 1: The Power of Shared Interests

Shared interests are activities or pursuits that human beings enjoy doing collectively. They can vary from sports, songs, art, and anything that brings people together with a common hobby. Pursuing shared pursuits is useful in several methods.

Shared hobbies create an experience of community

Shared interests provide a possibility for people to hook up with others who share comparable passions. It creates a feeling of belonging and network, that's important for our emotional and intellectual nicely-being. When humans percentage a common interest, they could engage in significant conversations and construct relationships that could final a lifetime.

Shared pastimes provide possibilities for growth and mastering
Pursuing shared hobbies may be an exquisite way to research new talents and make bigger our understanding. When we engage in sports with others who are captivated by identical things, we can study from each different, percentage understanding and abilities, and assist every different's growth.

Shared pursuits can lead to progressed physical and mental health
Participating in shared pursuits can high-quality city impact on our bodily and mental fitness. For example, accomplishing sports activities or other bodily sports can improve our fitness stages and decrease strain stages. Pursuing innovative pursuits, such as art or music, can also have a tremendous impact on our mental fitness by way of decreasing tension and melancholy.

Part 2: The Power of Shared Goals

Shared dreams are aspirations or objectives that human beings work towards collectively. They may be non-public or expert goals that require collaboration and teamwork. Pursuing shared goals will have several benefits.

Shared designs create an experience of purpose
Shared dreams offer people withfeelingeel of cause and direction. When human beings work closer to a commonplace purpose, they are motivated to take action and make progress toward achieving that intention. This sense of cause may be highly empowering and can assist people to conquer limitations and challenges.

Shared goals buriedeementwith and accountability
When human beingsntngs collectively toward a shared goal, they contend ruct agree with responsibility. They learn how to rely upon each other, talk efficaciously, and work collaboratively to gain their goals. This may be useful in non-public and professional relationships, as it could lingualingeel of team spirit and foster a supportive environment.

Shared desires can result in more fulfillment

When people paint collectively towards a shared intention, they could reap more success than they would personally. This is because they could leverage every different's strengths and abilities, share assets, and provide help and encouragement to each other. Working collectively in the direction of a shared intention can also result in new possibilities and growth, as people research every other and increase their understanding and capabilities.

Part 3: Growing Together: Combining Shared Interests and Shared Goals

When people integrate shared pastimes and shared dreams, they can revel in even extra blessings. Pursuing shared pursuits can create a sturdy basis for building relationships while pursuing shared dreams coffer course and purpose for those relationships. When mixed, they can create effective pressure for increase and development.

Combining shared pastimes and shared dreams creates a strong feeling of the network
When humans pursue shared hobbies and shared dreams, they invent a strong feeling of network. They percentage commonplace passions and targets, that may result in deep and significant relationships. This feeling of the community can be noticeably useful for our emotional and mental properly-being because it offers

CHAPTER 7 Weathering Life's Challenges:

Life is unpredictable, and challenges are a herbal part of it. Everyone faces problems at some unspecified time in the future of their lives. It may be whatever from economic hardships, health problems, relationship troubles, professional setbacks, or another surprising event that can shake us to our middle. However, how we cope with those demanding situations could make all the difference. Supporting every different thru difficult instances could make the adventure less lonely and overwhelming. It can offer hope, consolation, and the energy to overcome even the most difficult limitations. In this article, we can talk about ways to climate life's demanding situations and support every other via hard times.

Acknowledge the assignment:

The first step in coping with any task is to well know its life. Denying or ignoring the trouble could make it worse and tougher to triumph over. We want to just accept that we are going through an undertaking and that it could take time and effort to triumph over it. Once we've mentioned the hassle, we can begin searching out answers and support.

COMMUNICATE:

Communication is essential in terms of dealing with challenges. We want to speak to each differently, share our emotions, and ask for assistance if needed. Sometimes, just speaking approximately our issues can offer a few remedies and make us sense less alone. We must inspire open and sincere verbal exchange, wherein everybody feels secure to explicit their thoughts and feelings without judgment.

LISTEN:

Listening is simply as important as speaking. We need to listen actively and empathetically to each different. This means paying attention to what the opposite man or woman is saying, understanding their angle, and validating their emotions. Listening can help build trust, toughen relationships, and provide emotional guidance.

PROVIDE PRACTICAL HELP:

When going through an assignment, realistic help may be priceless. This can be something from cooking a meal, running errands, providing a trip, or assisting with family chores. Practical assistance can reduce strain, provide a few remedies, and allow the character to be cognizant of solving the hassle.

OFFER EMOTIONAL SUPPORT:

Emotional aid is equally crucial as sensible assistance. We need to offer encouragement, motivation, and a shoulder to lean on. Simple gestures together with sending a textual content message, giving a hug, or spending time with the character could make a big difference. Emotional help can raise morale, reduce anxiety, and provide hope.

BE POSITIVE:

Staying advantageous may be tough whilst dealing with a task, but it's far more important. We need to recognition at the matters we can manipulate, as opposed to the matters we cannot. We need to encourage every other to have a fine mindset, search for the silver lining, and locate reasons to be grateful. Being high quality can offer a sense of wish, reduce strain, and improve intellectual health.

Practice Self-Care:

Taking care of ourselves is crucial when dealing with a challenge. We want to prioritize self-care, inclusive of ingesting properly, getting sufficient sleep, workout often, and taking time to loosen up. Self-care can reduce stress, enhance physical fitness, and enhance our temper.

SEEK PROFESSIONAL HELP:

Sometimes, we may additionally need professional assistance to cope with a challenge. This will be anything from remedy, counseling, or medical treatment. We should inspire every other to search for assistance while wished, with no disgrace or stigma. Professional assistance can provide the equipment, guidance, and support wished to triumph over the assignment.

Life is full of demanding situations, and we can not always manipulate what occurs to us. However, we can manage how we reply to those demanding situations. Supporting every other thru difficult instances could make the journey less lonely and overwhelming. We need to acknowledge the assignment, talk openly, concentrate actively, offer sensible and emotional guidance, live effectively, exercise care sought to seek the right help when wanted. Together, we can weather life's demanding situations and emerge stronger and greater resilient.

CHAPTER 8 Cultivating Gratitude:

When it comes to cultivating a long-lasting courting, there are few things extra vital than gratitude. Appreciating every other can help construct a strong foundation of agree with and mutual respect, and it may make it less complicated to weather the ups and downs of lifestyles collectively. In this article, we're going to explore why cultivating gratitude is so important for relationships, and we're going to provide some recommendations for a way you may start incorporating greater appreciation into your relationship.

The Benefits of Gratitude in Relationships

There are many benefits to cultivating gratitude in relationships. Some of the most essential include:

Increased Trust and Respect: When you express gratitude and appreciation for your partner, you are displaying to them that you cost and appreciate them. This can assist construct a foundation of agreement and mutual appreciation, which is important for a hy and lasting dating.

Improved Communication: Expressing gratitude and appreciation can also enhance conversation in your relationship. When you're thankful for something your companion has carried out, it may be simpler to talk approximately your emotions and desires constructively.

Greater Emotional Intimacy: Gratitude also can assist domesticate more emotional intimacy in your dating. When you have a specific appreciation for your associate, you are displaying vulnerability and opening yourself up to a deeper emotional connection.

Reduced Conflict: When you are thankful for your companion, it could be easier to overlook minor annoyances or conflicts. Instead of focusing on the terrible, you may awareness of the fine components of your courting and work together to resolve any issues that do get up.

Increased Happiness: Finally, gratitude can virtually make you and your accomplice happier. When our awareness of the belongings you're thankful for in your courting, it let you respect and revel in every other extra fully.

How to Cultivate Gratitude in Your Relationship

Now that we have explored the advantages of cultivating gratitude in relationships, let's check a few sensible ways to do so:

Start Small: You don't have to make grand gestures to explicit gratitude and appreciation to your associate. Start with small matters, like announcing "thank you" while your partner does something kind or considerate.

Make it a Habit: Cultivating gratitude calls for exercise, so make it n everyday habit. Try to explicit appreciation for your companion at least once a day, whether or not it is in character, over the cellphone, or in a textual content message.

Focus on Specifics: When expressing gratitude, be unique approximately what you are thankful for. Instead of simply pronouncing "Thank you," try pronouncing "I respect the way you took care of the dishes remaining night. It made my night so much less difficult."

Be Mindful: To cultivate gratitude, it is vital to remember the things your partner does for you. Pay attention to small matters, like making your coffee in the morning or doing the laundry, and take time to acknowledge them.

Practice Active Listening: When your partner expresses gratitude or appreciation for something you have executed, take some time to concentrate and understand their words. This can assist deepen your emotional connection and construct acceptance as true.

Make it a Two-Way Street: Finally, keep in mind that gratitude should be a two-manner street. Express appreciation for your associate, however, additionally make an effort to be well-known and be thankful for the things they do for you.

Cultivating gratitude in n your relationship will have a profound effect on your happiness and nicely-being, in addition to the fitness of your dating. By expressing gratitude and appreciation for each different frequency, you can construct consideration and mutual respect, improve verbal exchange, and deepen your emotional connection. So begin small, make it a habit, and have in mind the many things your accomplice does for you every day. With time and practice, you may locate that cultivating gratitude comes certainly and will let you build a long-lasting

CHAPTER 9 The Culture of Instant:

In the modern-day tradition of instant gratification, it's smooth to fall into the trap of giving up on relationships when matters get hard. But for folks that are devoted to constructing a lasting and significant date, there are ways to stay on the path and overcome the demanding situations that stand up along the manner. Here are some effective guidelines for retaining a long-time period of dating in a tradition that values instant pride.

Build a robust basis: Before embarking on a protracted-term relationship, it is vital to ensure that the inspiration is robust. This method organizes mutual admiration, agreement, and conversation. Take time to get to recognize your companion, and share your mind and feelings as well. When there's a solid foundation of trust and appreciation, it's less complicated to climate the storms to necessarily come.

Set realistic expectancies: In a way of life that values immediate pride, it is clear to fall into the lure of watching for immediate gratification in all elements of lifestyles. However, on the subject of relationships, it is crucial to set realistic expectations. This means expertise that a wholesome courting takes time, effort, and endurance. Don't assume your associate to be best, and don't assume each second of your courting to be perfect either.

Focus on the effective: In any courting, there may be America and downs. When things get hard, it's easy to focus on the bad aspects of the relationship. However, it is essential to remember the fact that there are high-quality elements as nicely. Attempt to focus on the matters that you recognize approximately your accomplice and specify your gratitude often.

Communicate overtly and truly: Communication is the inspiration of any healthful relationship. When matters get difficult, it's crucial to speak brazenly and absolutely with your companion. This way sharing your thoughts and feelings, even though they're difficult to express. It also approaches listening to your accomplice's thoughts and emotions with an open mind.

Work together as a team: In any relationship, it is vital to work collectively as a crew. This way assisting every different via tough instances and celebrating every other's successes. It also approaches working collectively to overcome challenges and construct stronger relationships.

Prioritize the best time together: In a trendy busy world, it's smooth to let time along with your accomplice slip away. However, it's important to prioritize fine time together. This way place aside time to do matters which you each make attempting to attach emotionally regularly.

Practice forgiveness: No one is perfect, and errors can be made in any dating. When errors occur, it's crucial to exercise forgiveness. This means letting go of grudges and moving forward definitely.

Be an affected person: Building a healthful, long-term relationship takes time and endurance. Don't count on matters to show up overnight, and don't be discouraged if progress is gradual. Keep running at it, and consider that your efforts can pay off in the end.

Don't compare your dating to others: In a subculture that values instantaneous gratification, it's smooth to examine your dating to others. However, every relationship is unique, and evaluating yourself by others may be a recipe for sadness. Focus on your dating, and work to make it the first-rate it can be.

Take care of yourself: In any dating, it's critical to attend to yourself. This way look after your bodily, emotional, and intellectual fitness. When you're healthy and glad, you're higher capable of making contributions to a wholesome and glad dating.

Seek assistance when wished: Building a wholesome, lengthy-term relationship isn't continually clean. If you're suffering, don't be afraid to seek assistance. This may additionally suggest speaking to a therapist, searching for advice from a trusted buddy, or attending couples counseling.

Conclusions

The are 29 good steps listed to consider,
No Divorce Happy Home Forever

1, we view comfort in our responsibility as together until the end of time."

2. " Through various challenges, we found the mysterious fix to a blissful home: remaining together until the end of time."

3. " Our adoration is a rugged bond that keeps us joined together, guaranteeing a long period of harmony."

4. " With unfaltering devotion, we've opened the key to an upbeat home, liberated from the shadows of separation."

5. " Together perpetually, we stand as a demonstration of the force of affection, making an agreeable safe house inside our home."

6. " In the domain of never-ending love, our home stands tall, safe to the types of separation."

7. " Through chuckling and tears, we embrace the mystery of fellowship, cultivating a cheerful home that challenges us. " Our hearts thump as one, monitoring the key to a home based on adoration, perpetually safe from the danger of separation."

9. " Inside the walls of our home, the way to timeless satisfaction lives, protecting us from the tempest of separation."

10. " Inseparably, we set out on an excursion of never-ending love, defending our home from the aggravation of separation."

11 . " Joined by affection's hug, we open the key to an amicable home, a haven where separation can't intrude."

12. " In the domain of solid bonds, our home remains steadfast, perpetually getting away from the grip of separation."

13. " With adoration as our establishment, we have deciphered the code to a happy home, distant by the strife of separation."

14. " Together everlasting, our adoration blooms, sustaining a shelter where separation dare not track."

15. " Inside our souls, we convey the way into a happy home, joined in an adoration that safeguards us from being separate. " Through responsibility and empathy, we've found the key to a home spilling over with satisfaction, ruling out separate."

17. " Like two spirits entwined, we dance to the musicality of everlasting, challenging the chances and banishing divorce from our home."

18. " With immovable dedication, we've opened the key to a home loaded up with chuckling and love, impenetrable to separate."

19. " Our romantic tale is carved in the walls of our home, an unwritten pronouncement that precludes separate from its consecrated grounds."
20. " In the embroidery of harmony, we have woven a haven, where separation is nevertheless ancient history."
21. " With hearts weaved, we've found the key to a home that emanates satisfaction, perpetually protected from the shadows of separation."
22. " In the orchestra of our adoration, the notes perpetually resound, making a song that overwhelms the murmurs of separation."
23. " Limited by a rugged commitment, we've found the key to a home that flourishes, safe to the breaks of separation."
24. " Our affection is a stronghold, shielding our home from the invasion of separation, guaranteeing we stand up until the end of time."
25. " Inside the walls of our home, the key to never-ending satisfaction lives, bracing us against the dangers of separation."
26. " Through shared dreams and unfaltering help, we've opened the key to a home where separation is nevertheless a far-off plausibility."
27. " Like two stars in the night sky, we sparkle brilliantly, enlightening a way to a home immaculate by the dimness of separation."

28. "In the nursery of affection, we've found the key to a prospering home, where separation will go away from undesirable weeds."
29. " As time passes, our adoration develops further, developing a home that separation can't enter."

Thanks for reading this wonderful book and more importantly thanks for getting this book may your HOME be blessed